Keto Diet Cookbook

Low-Carb High-Fat Recipes for Men and Women

By Nugahana KTN

Table of content

Introduction

Congratulations on purchasing this book, *Keto Diet Cookbook, Low-Carb High-Fat Recipes for Men and Women.* Thank you for doing so.

When it comes to ketogenic diet, people always have questions like what effects it will have on your body, how to compensate for various factors in life, and how to have success with it. The questions can be endless.

The chapters in this book will serve as a guide to answer the most pressing questions about keto. We will address the most pressing concerns from our observation for someone who is interested in keto.

Once we get through all the basics of what keto is and how it works, we'll dive deep into some of the most delicious recipes that the ketogenic diet has to offer. If you are someone who loves a lot of flavor or someone who enjoys the sweeter things in life, we've got some amazing recipes that will soon be staples in your kitchen!

There are so many books on this subject on the market but I am glad you choose this one. Once again, thanks for choosing this one! We have put in all our efforts to ensure that it is full of so much useful information. please enjoy it!

What is the Keto Diet?

In very simple terms, the keto diet is a low-carb diet that aims to shift the way your body processes the food that you eat. Your body typically thrives on the carbohydrates that you eat and it in turn uses those carbohydrates the boost up your blood sugar. The only problem this boost poses is that *what goes up, must come down!*

When you start on keto, what you're doing is cutting your carbohydrates down to only 5% of your daily macronutrient intake. It will also have a maximum limit of 20 grams per day. It's also very important to track what you're taking into your body for first few weeks to get a mastery of how this works.

The aim of keto is to shift your body from running on carbohydrates to running on healthy fats and a very specific amount of protein. By you giving your body calculated measurements and percentages of carbs, fats, and proteins, your body is forced to run only on the fat that you're giving it. With time your body will learn to live just on the fat you give it and what it had stored over the years. So many of us have huge stores of stubborn fat that has denied to go and won't leave us irrespective of what we do. Do you know what to do with these kinds of fat? The answer is to give your body no choice but to burn that fat to keep going!

What are the Advantages of keto?

By giving your body more of healthier fats like avocados, coconut oil, and nuts, you are giving your body an alternative source of fuel. This will cause your body to shifts over to a different mode of metabolism. Your body will now be in a state of constant fat burning. This is easy because your body has fat stores that it burns and use as fuel to drive you.

Most of us have huge fat stores that we are trying to get rid of but we don't know that if you teach your body, this will be a huge fuel source that it can use to run on *always*. This can lead to so much more energy in your body and muscles than you had before. You will discover that when your body starts burning its's fat, fat loss comes to you with far less effort than you realized was possible

Many who have tried keto have seen and can testify to the fact that it makes drastic changes not only to their quality of life, but also to their health, the clarity of their skin, and even the resolution and improvement of severe physical maladies like type II diabetes!

Things to Keep in Mind

When it comes to keto one of the biggest misconceptions is that all fat is created equal. This like we will see shortly is not true. When you want to start keto, you would want to take into account the types of fats you're eating. This is important because you will know that you're giving your body exactly what it needs to thrive, repair, and keep going.

You need to also remember that *keto is not a high-protein diet*. It's a low-carb, high-fat diet that relies on a specific balance between fat, protein, and carbohydrates to give your body the best fat burning possible. Truth is your body needs protein but in excess it could be a setback in your weight loss progress.

When you're on keto, your body purges a large amount of your body's stored electrolytes. It's important for you to drink plenty of water throughout the day (yes, I'm sorry, you're going to be peeing *all the time*). This ensure that you don't feel run-down, tired, or dehydrated while you're doing keto!

Breakfast

The keto diet has gained a lot of room among our classic breakfast foods like eggs, but you need to know that keto breakfast doesn't have to stick to the same boring routine of breakfast. If you're not an ovo-vegetarian we've got you covered. We know that breakfast is even more of a conundrum but we're looking out for you by including some protein-rich, egg-free breakfast dishes. These recipes below will give you new twists on old favorites so you can start every new day in a keto way.

Egg Scramble

Servings: 6

Time Required: About 4.5 hours

Ingredients:

- 1 onion, diced
- 2 cups cheddar cheese, grated
- 10 eggs
- 1 cup whole milk
- 1 tsp. salt
- 1 tsp. pepper

Directions:

1. Put the diced onion and cheese into a clean empty slow cooker.
2. In a clean empty mixing bowl, whisk together the milk and eggs until the eggs are beaten and form a good mixture with the milk. Add the salt and the pepper and stir to mixture till it mixes thoroughly.
3. Poor the egg mixture obtained over the ingredients in a clean empty slow cooker.
4. Cover the pot and cook its content on low heat for 4 hours.
5. Serve hot and enjoy.

Pressure Cooker Soft-Boiled Eggs

Servings: 6

Time Required: About 10 minutes

Ingredients:

- 6 large eggs
- ¾ cup water

Directions:

- Place the steamer rack into your pressure cooker and pour in the water.
- Carefully place the eggs, still in the shell, on top of the steamer rack.
- Cover and lock the pot firmly.
- Using the Steam function, set the cook time to 2 minutes and let cook.
- When the cook time is up, remove the eggs and serve hot.

Keto Hot Breakfast Cereal

Servings: 1

Time Required: About 10 minutes

Ingredients:

- 2 Tbsp. coconut flour
- 3 Tbsp. golden flaxseed meal
- 1 ½ cups unsweetened almond milk
- Sugar-free sweetener to taste

Directions:

1. In a clean empty bowl mix together the coconut flour and flaxseed meal.
2. Add the obtained mixture to an empty small sauce pan and stir in the almond milk. Cook over medium heat until it begins to thicken.
3. Once the mixture in the pan has begun to thicken, stir in the sweetener to taste (approximately ½ tsp.).
4. Serve Hot and enjoy

Omelets in a Cup

Servings: 4

Time Required: About 20 minutes

Ingredients:

- 4 eggs
- ½ cup onion, diced
- ½ cup bell pepper, diced
- ½ cup cheddar cheese, grated
- ¼ cup half and half

Directions:

1. In a clean empty mixing bowl, whisk together all ingredients until the eggs are well beaten and everything is well mixed and combined. Season with some salt and pepper.

2. Divide the mixture obtained into four small canning jars. Loosely screw the lids onto the jars.

3. Place a clean empty steamer rack in a double boiler/steamer and pour 2 cups water into the pot.

4. Place the jars containing the mixture on the steamer rack and cover the pot.

5. Bring water to a boil and let to steam for 10 minutes.

6. Remove the jars from the pot and serve the eggs in the jars.

Cauliflower Waffles

Servings: 1

Time Required: About 25 minutes

Ingredients:

- ½ large head cauliflower, riced
- 1 cup mozzarella cheese, finely shredded
- 1 cup collard greens
- 1/3 cup Parmesan cheese
- 2 large eggs
- 2 stalks green onion
- 1 Tbsp. sesame seeds
- 1 Tbsp. olive oil
- 2 tsp. fresh chopped thyme
- 1 tsp. garlic powder
- ½ tsp. ground black pepper
- ½ teaspoon salt

Directions:

1. Cut out the cauliflower into its florets, slice the spring onion into reasonable sizes and pull the thyme leaves from their stems.

2. Chop the cauliflower florets in a food processor, using the pulse mode until the floret are ground into a coarse, crumbly texture.

3. Add the spring onion, thyme and collard greens to the food processor and continue pulsing until everything is thoroughly mixed and well combined.

4. Transfer the content from the food processor into to a large mixing bowl.

5. To the content in the bowl, add the mozzarella cheese, Parmesan cheese, eggs, sesame seeds, olive oil, garlic powder, black pepper, and salt.

6. Mix all the above till it forms a loose batter.

7. Preheat a waffle iron till it is red hot, and when the iron is red hot, spoon in the batter. Cook until the waffles are beginning to brown.

8. Serve hot and enjoy.

Flax Seed Cereal

Servings: 6

Time Required: About 90 minutes

Ingredients:

- ½ cup milled flax seed
- ½ cup hulled hemp seeds
- 2 Tbsp. ground cinnamon
- ½ cup apple juice
- 1 Tbsp. coconut oil

Directions:

1. Preheat oven to about 300 degrees Fahrenheit.
2. Combine the dry ingredients in a blender or food processor. Add apple juice and coconut oil and blend until the mixture is thoroughly blended and moderately smooth.
3. Spread the batter about 1/16-inch thick on a parchment-lined baking sheet.
4. Place the content in the oven and bake on the oven's center rack for 15 minutes. Reduce the heat of the oven to about 250 degrees and bake for another 10 minutes.
5. Remove the baking sheet from the oven. Cut the baked cereal into ½-inch squares or of a size you desire. A pizza cutter works well for this.
6. Return the baking sheet to the oven and turn off the heat. Keep the sheet in the oven with the door closed for about an hour. At this point, the cereal should be nice and crisp.
7. Serve with almond milk or other non-dairy milk and enjoy.

Mini Mushroom Keto Quiche

Servings: 6

Time Required: About 20 minutes

Ingredients:

- ½ cup Swiss cheese, grated
- ¼ cup fresh mushrooms, chopped
- ¼ cup spring onion, diced
- 4 eggs
- ¼ cup milk
- 1 cup water

Directions:

1. Using a silicone or heat-proof egg tray, divide the cheese evenly between the cups in the tray. You can achieve this by pressing the cheese into the bottom of the cups.
2. Divide the mushrooms and onions among the cups, placing them on top of the cheese in the cups.
3. Crack the eggs into a food processor or blender. Season the eggs with salt and pepper. Blend the mixture until the ingredients are well combined and smooth. Pour the mixture obtained into the cups on top of the cheese, mushrooms and onions.
4. Place the cups into a steamer rack in a steamer pot and add the water.
5. Carefully place the tray on top of the steamer rack and cover the pot.
6. Bring the water to a boil and let steam the food for 15 minutes.
7. After a few minutes of cooling, pop the mini quiches out of the tray and serve immediately.

Egg Crepes

Servings: 4

Time Required: About 15 minutes

Ingredients:

- 6 eggs
- 5 gms. cream cheese, softened
- 1 tsp. cinnamon
- 1 Tbsp. sugar-free sweetener
- 1 Tbsp. butter (for sautéing)

Filling ingredients:

- 8 Tbsp. butter, softened
- 1/3 cup sugar-free sweetener
- 1 Tbsp. cinnamon

Directions:

1. Blend the first four ingredients together in a blender until the mixture is smooth and well combined. Let the batter rest for 5 minutes.
2. Heat 1 tablespoon of butter in a nonstick pan on medium heat.
3. Pour the obtained batter into the pan to form a thin layer of about 6 inches in diameter. Cook this batter for about 2 minutes, then flip sides and cook for an additional minute.
4. Remove the crepe and place on a warm plate. Repeat until the batter is gone. It should yield about 8 crepes.
5. Mix sweetener and some cinnamon in a small bowl.
6. Stir half of the obtained mixture into the softened butter until it is smooth.
7. Spread 1 tablespoon of the mixture onto the center of each crepe.

8. Roll up the crepe and sprinkle it with the sweetener and cinnamon mixture.

9. Serve hot and enjoy

Keto Breakfast Sandwich

Ingredients:

¼ medium avocado, sliced

¼-1/2 tsp. chili sauce (to taste)

1 egg, beaten

1 tablespoon cream cheese

2 sausage patties

2 tablespoons sharp cheddar

Sea salt & pepper to taste

Directions:

1. Over medium heat, warm a clean empty skillet and prepare the sausage patties

2. Add the shredded cheddar cheese and the cream cheese in a small bowl, then heat the mixture in the microwave for 20-30 seconds while stirring till it melts.

3. Add the chili sauce, if needed, to cheese mixture and stir until it is mixed.

4. Scramble the egg in a small bowl and add desired seasonings. Add salt and pepper to taste. Cook to make an omelet or a manageable shape and add to the sandwich.

5. Using one sausage patty as the bottom "bun," layer egg, cheese mixture, and avocado in an order that is satisfactory for you, then top with second patty.

6. Slice if desired and enjoy!

Egg Cups with Hash

Yield: 3 servings

Serving Size: 2 cups

Prep Time: 10 min.

Cook Time: 25 min.

Ingredients:

¼ c. mayonnaise

¼ c. parmesan cheese, grated

¼ c. yellow onion, diced

1 ½ c. ham, diced

1 clove fresh garlic, minced

2 tsp. fresh parsley, chopped

3 tbsp. almond flour

6 large eggs

Sea salt & pepper to taste

Directions:

1. Preheat oven to 375° Fahrenheit and coat a muffin tin with non-stick spray or preferred fat source.

2. In a clean empty food processor, lightly grind the onion, parsley, ham, and garlic until a coarse grind is achieved.

3. Into your mixture, stir the cheese, mayonnaise, and flour along with salt and pepper until thoroughly incorporated.

4. Put the mixture into 6 of the cups in the muffin tin, taking care to press it down so it fills all the edges.

5. Bake the obtained mixture for five minutes, then take back out of the oven.

6. Crack one egg into each of the cups, breaking the yolks if you prefer to do so.

7. Bake again at 375° Fahrenheit for 20 minutes, or until the egg is fully cooked.

8. Let stand for 5 minutes to cool a bit, then pop cups out of the muffin tin.

9. Serve hot and enjoy!

Carrot Cake Pancakes

Yield: 8 servings

Serving Size: 1 pancake

Prep Time: 10 min.

Cook Time: 20 min.

Ingredients:

¼ c. almond milk, unsweetened

½ tsp. apple cider vinegar

¾ c. almond flour

1 ½ tsp. baking powder

1 tsp. cinnamon

1/3 c. carrots, grated

2 lg. eggs

2 tbsp. chopped pecans

2 tbsp. coconut flour

3 tbsp. monk fruit sweetener or preferred sweetener

Directions:

1. In a clean empty mixing bowl, mix eggs, almond milk, and vinegar with a whisk until smooth.

2. Add some flours, sweetener, baking powder, cinnamon, and a pinch of salt to the mixture and whisk until its smooth.

3. Heat a clean skillet over medium heat and let pan get hot.

4. Fold in the carrots and nuts and set aside and add butter or oil to the pan to prevent sticking.

5. Spoon mixture into the pan, about ¼ cup at a time.

6. Cook for two to three minutes on each side of the pancake, or until bubbles form on the edges.

7. Cook until firm and then transfer to a plate.

8. Serve topped with cream cheese or sugar-free maple syrup!

Baked Eggs with Chorizo

Yield: 3 servings

Serving Size: 1 large wedge

Prep Time: 15 min.

Cook Time: 20 min.

Ingredients:

½ tsp. paprika

¾ c. shredded pepper jack cheese

1 pinch cayenne pepper (optional)

1 sm. avocado, chopped

3 oz. chorizo sausage, ground

3 tbsp. sour cream

5 lg. eggs

Sea salt & pepper to taste

Directions:

1. Preheat oven to 400° Fahrenheit.

2. Heat an oven-safe skillet over medium heat and cook the chorizo for eight to ten minutes or until fully cooked through.

3. Put chorizo aside in a bowl and return the pan to the heat, keeping the chorizo drippings in the pan.

4. Once the pan is returned to sufficient heat, crack the eggs into the pan, seasoning with salt and pepper to taste.

5. Sprinkle chorizo back into the pan and top with cayenne, paprika, and cheese.

6. Bake at 400° Fahrenheit for 15-20 minutes, or until it is done to your liking and the cheese is bubbly.

7. Let stand for five minutes or so before slicing into thirds.

8. Serve topped with sour cream and avocado!

Soft Boiled Eggs with Herbs

Yield: 1 serving

Serving Size: 3 eggs

Prep Time: 5 min.

Cook Time: 6 min.

Ingredients:

3 lg. eggs

1 tbsp. butter, melted

¼ tsp. fresh basil, chopped

¼ tsp. fresh thyme, chopped

Sea salt & pepper

Directions:

1. Fill a medium saucepan halfway with water and heat it till it boils.

2. Carefully place the eggs into the water, taking care not to break the egg shells.

3. For six minutes, boil the eggs, then remove from the hot water.

4. Remove the eggs from the boiling water, then run under some cold water to halt the cooking process.

5. Peel the shells from the eggs and rinse well to remove any remnants of the shell.

6. In a bowl, place the eggs then drizzle with the butter. Top with the herbs, salt, and pepper and enjoy!

Ham and Cheese Soufflés

Yield: 4 servings

Serving Size: 1 soufflé

Prep Time: 10 min.

Cook Time: 22 min.

Ingredients:

½ c. heavy cream

1 c. cheddar cheese, shredded

1 sm. yellow onion, diced

2 cloves fresh garlic, minced

2 tbsp. fresh chives, chopped

2 tbsp. olive oil

6 lg. eggs

6 oz. ham, diced

Sea salt & pepper to taste

Directions:

1. Preheat the oven to 400° Fahrenheit and grease ramekins or baking dishes with non-stick spray or some other preferred source of fat.

2. In a clean empty skillet over medium heat, pour the olive oil and let to warm.

3. Cook the onion for about five minutes, or until they begin to become translucent. Also add garlic and cook for about a minute more.

4. In a mixing bowl, combine all the remaining ingredients and mix until fully mixed.

5. Add the onions and garlic to the mixing bowl, mix, then pour into baking dishes.

6. Bake for 18 to 22 minutes or until the egg is cooked all the way through.

7. Allow to cool for about five minutes before serving and enjoy!

Lunch

Meat, poultry and fish are a major part of most keto diets. The recipes in this section of the book include the main dishes, vegetable side dishes and some desserts. For the lunch recipes, we've focused on dishes that are light, easy enough to prepare and simple that they'll fit perfectly into your mid-day routine. These meals also aren't deficient in flavor. They're also interesting enough that they can be used as dinner or part of dinner, if you decide to prepare them a little later in the day.

Tomato Parm Salad

Yield: 4 servings

Serving Size: 1 bowl

Prep Time: 10 min.

Ingredients:

¼ c. lemon juice, fresh

½ sm. red onion, thinly sliced

1 tbsp. dill, fresh & chopped

1 tbsp. white wine vinegar

1/3 c. extra virgin olive oil

2 oz. fresh mozzarella, chopped

2 tbsp. basil, fresh & chopped

2 tbsp. cilantro, fresh & chopped

6 med. Roma tomatoes, chopped

Fresh parmesan, grated

Sea salt & pepper to taste

Directions:

1. In a clean empty small bowl, whisk together the oil, lemon juice, vinegar, and herbs.

2. In a clean empty large bowl, combine the tomatoes, onions, mozzarella, salt and pepper to taste, and dressing.

3. Toss to coat all ingredients thoroughly in the dressing.

4. Cover and keep chilled until ready to serve. Serve garnished with freshly grated parmesan.

Deviled Egg Salad

Yield: 6 servings

Serving Size: ¾ cup

Prep Time: 15 min.

Cook Time: 10 min.

Ingredients:

½ sm. red pepper, diced

½ tsp. hot sauce (optional)

½ tsp. paprika

1 med. stalk celery, diced

1 tbsp. apple cider vinegar

12 lg. eggs, hardboiled

2 green onions, thinly sliced

2 tbsp. Dijon mustard

6 tbsp. mayonnaise

Sea salt & pepper to taste

Directions:

1. Hard boil your eggs. When ready, peel, and set aside.

2. In a clean empty small bowl, whisk together mayonnaise, vinegar, hot sauce, mustard, and paprika to form your dressing.

3. Chop the hardboiled eggs into bite-sized pieces and place in a clean empty large bowl.

4. Add green onion, celery, and pepper to the bowl and top with dressing. Toss to coat.

5. Season with salt and pepper to taste. Serve chilled and enjoy!

Classic Egg Salad

Yield: 4 servings

Serving Size: ½ cup

Prep Time: 10 min.

Cook Time: 15 min.

Ingredients:

¾ c. mayonnaise

1 ½ tsp. yellow mustard

2 med. green onions, thinly sliced

2 med. stalks celery, sliced

8 lg. eggs, hardboiled

Sea salt & pepper to taste

Directions:

1. Hard boil your eggs. When it is ready, peel, and set aside.

2. Chop the eggs into bite sizes and add to a medium size mixing bowl. Garnish with celery and onion.

3. Add mayonnaise, salt, mustard, and pepper to the bowl and stir until well combined.

Garden Salad with Creamy Buttermilk Dressing

Yield: 3 servings

Serving Size: 2 cups

Prep Time: 10 min.

Ingredients:

½ c. cherry tomatoes, halved

½ tsp. onion powder

1 to 2 tbsp. buttermilk

1 tsp. parsley, dried

2 tbsp. mayonnaise

2 tbsp. sour cream

3 lg. eggs, hardboiled

3 oz. cheddar cheese, shredded

3 oz. deli-sliced turkey

4 ½ c. romaine lettuce, roughly chopped

Directions:

1. In a clean empty small bowl, whisk together the sour cream, mayonnaise, onion powder, and parsley.

2. Add some buttermilk, whisking constantly until it is thin and smooth. Gauge the texture and thickness of the dressing as you go an add more or less buttermilk as is needed.

3. In three salad clean empty bowls, separate the romaine.

4. Top with other ingredients and drizzle with two tablespoons of dressing each.

5. Serve cold and enjoy!

Bagel-Wrapped Links

Yield: 8 servings

Serving Size: 1 link

Prep Time: 15 min.

Cook Time: 15 min.

Ingredients:

¼ tsp. garlic powder

½ c. cheddar cheese, shredded

1 ¼ c. almond flour

1 ½ c. mozzarella cheese, shredded

1 lg. egg

1 lg. egg white, beaten

2 oz. cream cheese, softened

2 tbsp. coconut flour

8 all-beef hotdogs

Directions:

1. Preheat the oven to 400° Fahrenheit and line a baking sheet with parchment paper.

2. In a microwave-safe bowl, combine cream cheese and mozzarella. Heat the mixture for 1 ½ minutes.

3. Remove the obtained mixture from the microwave, stir thoroughly and return to microwave for another 30 seconds if more melting is needed.

4. Pour the cheese mixture into the food processor along with the egg and blend it smooth.

5. Add flours and garlic powder to the food processor, allowing a sticky dough to form.

6. On a piece of plastic wrap, place the dough and wrap tightly. Set the dough to chill in the freezer until the oven is fully preheated or for at least 10 minutes.

7. Cut the ball of dough into 8 pieces and roll each piece into its own ball.

8. Roll each ball into a long thread about a foot long.

9. Wind the dough around each hotdog and press the seams closed with your thumb

10. Place all hotdogs on the baking sheet and sprinkle with cheddar cheese.

11. Bake for 12-15 minutes or until the dough is golden brown and cooked through.

12. Let cool for a couple of moments, then serve hot!

Roasted Pumpkin & Crisp Parmesan

Yield: 4 servings

Serving Size: 8 oz.

Prep Time: 10 min.

Cook Time: 20 min.

Ingredients:

¼ tsp. black pepper, ground

½ c. almonds, chopped

½ c. parsley, fresh & chopped

1 c. parmesan, freshly grated

1 sm. pumpkin (roughly 2 lbs.)

12 tsp. sea salt

2 tsp. thyme, dried

4 leaves sage, fresh & chopped

4 tbsp. extra virgin olive oil

Directions:

1. Hollow out the pumpkin and peel away all the outer skin using a vegetable peeler.

2. Preheat the oven to 400° Fahrenheit and line a baking sheet with foil.

3. Slice the pumpkin into reasonable wedges, about one inch thick.

4. Sprinkle some salt and pepper onto the wedges and place in the oven for about 20 minutes.

5. Remove cooked pumpkin from the oven and top with thyme, sage, and parsley. Toss lightly so it coats well if needed.

6. Sprinkle the almonds evenly over the pan, then follow with the parmesan.

7. Put the baking sheet under the broiler for about a minute, to allow the cheese to melt or put it back into the oven for up to five minutes so the cheese melts.

8. Serve hot and enjoy!

Curry Soup

Yield: 4 servings

Serving Size: 1 bowl

Prep Time: 25 min.

Cook Time: 20 min.

Ingredients:

¼ c. pumpkin seeds, raw

½ tsp. garlic powder

½ tsp. paprika

½ tsp. sea salt

¾ tsp. cumin

1 c. coconut milk, unsweetened

1 clove garlic, minced

1 med. onion, diced

2 c. carrots, chopped

2 tbsp. curry powder

3 c. cauliflower, riced

3 tbsp. extra virgin olive oil, divided

4 c. kale, chopped

4 c. vegetable broth

Sea salt & pepper to taste

Directions:

1. Heat a large sauté pan over medium heat with 2 tablespoons of olive oil. Once the oil is hot, add the rice cauliflower to the pan along with the

curry powder, cumin, salt, paprika, and garlic powder. Stir thoroughly to combine well.

2. While cooking, stir occasionally. Once the cauliflower is warmed through, remove it from the heat and keep in a bowl.

3. In a large clean empty pot over medium heat, add the remainder of your olive oil. Once it's hot, add the onion and allow it to cook for about four minutes. Add the garlic, then cook for about another two minutes.

4. To the large pot, add the broth, kale, carrots, and cauliflower. Stir to thoroughly incorporate.

5. Allow the mixture to come to a boil, drop the heat to low, and allow the soup to simmer for about 15 minutes.

6. Stir the coconut milk into the mixture along with salt and pepper to taste.

7. Garnish with pumpkin seeds and serve hot!

Broccoli Salad

Yield: 5 servings

Serving Size: 1 bowl

Prep Time: 15 min.

Cook Time: 10 min.

Ingredients:

5 slices bacon, chopped

1 lb. broccoli, chopped

½ c. cheddar cheese, shredded

¾ c. mayonnaise

¼ c. sour cream

1 tbsp. apple cider vinegar

1 tbsp. erythritol, or comparable measure of your preferred sweetener

¼ c. sunflower seeds

Directions:

1. Heat a clean empty large skillet over medium heat and cook the bacon until slightly crisp. Lay the bacon out on a paper towel to remove excess grease.

2. In a large clean empty mixing bowl, combine most (not all) of the bacon, broccoli, and shredded cheddar cheese. Toss to mix completely.

3. In a clean empty small bowl, combine mayonnaise, vinegar, sour cream, and sweetener.

4. Drizzle dressing over the larger mixing bowl and toss to coat all ingredients in the dressing.

5. Cover the mixing bowl and chill for about one hour.

6. Serve chilled and garnished with sunflower seeds and extra bacon!

Spicy Mushrooms

Servings: 2

Time Required: About 20 minutes

Ingredients:

- 8 grms. white mushrooms, chopped
- 2 large chili peppers, such as guajillo, poblano or New Mexico, seeded and chopped
- 1 tsp. olive oil
- 1 onion, chopped
- 6 cloves garlic, minced
- 1 tsp. ground cumin
- ½ tsp. dried oregano
- ½ tsp. smoked paprika
- ¼ tsp. ground cinnamon
- ¼ tsp. salt
- ¼ cup water
- 1 tsp. cider vinegar

Directions:

1. Heat the oil in a clean large empty skillet over medium heat. When the oil is really hot, add the onions to the pan and sauté until soft and translucent. Do this for about 5 minutes.
2. Add the garlic to the pan and sauté for one minute more.
3. Add mushrooms to the skillet and cook for 5 minutes more.
4. Transfer half of the onion and garlic to a clean blender or food processor.

5. Also add the chilis to the blender or food processor. Add cumin, oregano, paprika, cinnamon, salt and water. Blend until all of them are smooth.

6. Transfer the blended sauce mixture to the skillet and let them all cook until the sauce is heated through and bubbly. Do this for about 5 minutes.

7. Serve the mushrooms hot with steamed cauliflower and enjoy.

Herby Zucchini Noodles

Servings: 2

Time Required: About 20 minutes

Ingredients:

- 3 medium zucchini
- ½ tsp. salt
- ½ avocado
- 1 cup fresh basil leaves
- ¼ cup walnuts
- 2 cloves garlic
- ½ lemon
- ¼ cup Parmesan cheese, grated
- 1 Tbsp. olive oil
- Salt and pepper to taste

Directions:

1. Using a very sharp vegetable peeler, cut the zucchini into very thin ribbons. Use only the skin and outer flesh of the zucchini.
2. Toss the zucchini with salt in a colander and set aside for the salt to penetrate the zucchini.
3. Place the pealed avocado, basil, walnuts, garlic, lemon, and cheese in blender or food processor and pulse until the content is smooth. Add a few drops of water to adjust the consistency if necessary.
4. Heat 1 tablespoon of olive oil in a skillet over medium heat.
5. Sauté the zucchini until it begins to soften. Do this for about 3-5 minutes and transfer result to a mixing bowl.

6. Gently toss the zucchini with the dressing until all are well coated and enjoy

Keto Deviled Eggs

Servings: 4

Time Required: 15 minutes

Ingredients:

- 8 eggs
- ¼ cup mayonnaise
- 2 tsp. mustard
- 1 tsp. lemon juice
- 1 tsp. smoked paprika
- Salt and pepper

Directions:

1. Hard boil the eggs, peel and then slice in half lengthwise.
2. Slice in half lengthwise.
3. Carefully remove the egg yolks from the whites. In a medium bowl, use a fork to mash the yolks with mayonnaise, mustard, vinegar, salt and pepper to taste.
4. Carefully spoon the yolk mixture back into the hollows in the egg whited.
5. Sprinkle with smoked paprika.

Cheesy Cauliflower Nuggets

Servings: 4

Time Required: About 25 minutes

Ingredients:

- 1 medium cauliflower, riced
- 1 ½ cups cheddar cheese, shredded
- 3 eggs
- 2 tsp. paprika
- 1 tsp. turmeric
- ¾ tsp. rosemary

Directions:

1. If you're starting out with a whole head of cauliflower, then carefully clean it and chop it into florets. Place the obtained florets into a food processor and pulse until the cauliflower has the consistency of grains of rice. Alternatively, you can purchase pre-riced cauliflower.

2. Place cauliflower into a clean empty microwave safe bowl, and place in the microwave for 5-7 minutes.

3. Remove cauliflower from the oven and carefully place the cauliflower on a double layer of paper towel and cover with another double layer. Firmly press on the cauliflower in the paper towel to extract as much moisture from it as you can.

4. Transfer the pressed cauliflower to a clean empty medium mixing bowl. Add eggs one at a time, and then add the cheese to the bowl and mix.

5. Add the seasoning ingredients and then mix everything thoroughly with a wooden spoon or your hands till it is well mixed.

6. Heat the oils in a skillet over medium-high heat.

7. Form the cauliflower into 1-inch balls and then flatten them slight in your palm.

8. Place the cauliflower nuggets into the hot oil and fry until they're crispy on the bottom, about 2 minutes. Flip them and fry until the other side is crispy.

9. Serve hot and enjoy.

Keto Egg Salad

Servings: 8-10

Time Required: About 25 minutes

Ingredients:

- 10 eggs
- 2 Tbsp. mayonnaise
- 1 tsp. Dijon mustard
- ¼ tsp. smoked paprika
- 1 spring onion, diced
- Salt and pepper to taste

Directions:

1. Place the eggs in a clean large empty pot. Pour cold water until the eggs are completely covered. Heat the water till it boils for about 8-10 minutes. Remove them and cool them quickly by placing in cold water.

2. Peel of the egg shells and transfer them to a clean cutting board. Chop the eggs coarsely and transfer to a clean mixing bowl.

3. Add the rest of the ingredients to the mixing bowl and toss well to combine.

4. Serve garnished with chopped chives and enjoy.

Cheesy Vegetable Dip

Servings: 6

Time Required: About 35 minutes

Ingredients:

- 1 can (14 oz.) hearts of palm, drained
- 3 green onions, chopped
- ¼ cup mayonnaise
- 2 Tbsp. Italian seasoning
- ½ cup Parmesan cheese, grated
- 2 large eggs

Directions:

1. Pre-heat oven to 350 degrees Fahrenheit.
2. Lightly coat a small baking dish with cooking oil spray or butter.
3. Add all the ingredients, excluding the eggs, to a food processor or blender and pulse until the mixture is well-combined.
4. Add the eggs to the mixture and pulse again briefly, just enough to combine the egg with the other contents.
5. Spoon the dip into the oiled baking dish and bake for 15-20 minutes. Do this until the dip starts to bubble.
6. Carefully stir the dip for it to cook well and sprinkle the top with a bit more Parmesan cheese.
7. Return to the oven and bake until the top is beginning to brown. Do this for about 10 minutes more.
8. Serve hot and enjoy

Dinner Recipes

For most people, dinner is the main meal of the day and for the main meal of the day, you're going to want something as substantial as it is delicious. These recipes fit totally fine into that loop. We've brought together an irresistible collection of delicious main dishes, and appetizers that can work together in combination for a feast or your quick weeknight dinner.

Chicken Bacon Ranch Casserole

Yield: 8 servings

Serving Size: 1 square

Prep Time: 15 min.

Cook Time: 35 minutes

Ingredients:

¼ c. yellow onion, diced

½ c. sour cream

1 ½ lbs. chicken thighs, cooked & chopped

1 c. mayonnaise

1 lb. broccoli, chopped

1 tbsp. parsley, fresh & chopped

2 c. cheddar cheese, shredded & divided

2 tsp. garlic powder

4 slices bacon, chopped

8 oz. cream cheese, softened

Sea salt & pepper to taste

Directions:

1. Preheat the oven to 350° Fahrenheit and grease a baking dish with non-stick spray or your preferred fat source.

2. Add about an inch of water to a large clean empty saucepan and lower a steamer insert or metal strainer into it.

3. Toss the broccoli into the steamer and heat the water till it boils for about eight minutes or until when the broccoli is tender.

4. Drain out the excess moisture from the broccoli and set aside.

5. In a large clean empty mixing bowl, combine the mayonnaise, sour cream, and cream cheese.

6. Into the mixing bowl, add the parsley, salt, pepper, and garlic powder. Using a whisk or a fork, beat the mixture until smooth and well mixed.

7. Toss the broccoli, chicken, onion, half of the chopped bacon and 1 ½ cups of shredded cheese to the bowl and fold it in completely.

8. Pour the mixture into the baking dish and press into an even layer.

9. Top the casserole with the remaining cheese and bacon

10. Bake for 35 minutes or until the cheese is bubbling.

Lettuce-Wrapped Sloppy Joes

Yield: 4 servings

Serving Size: 2 wraps

Prep Time: 15 min.

Cook Time: 20 min.

Ingredients:

¼ c. tomato paste

½ head Boston or butter lettuce, leaves pulled off
1 lb. ground beef

¾ c. beef broth

1 med. stalk celery, diced

1 sm. yellow onion, diced

1 tsp. Dijon mustard

2 cloves garlic, minced

2 tbsp. erythritol sweetener or comparable amount of desired sweetener

2 tsp. Worcestershire sauce

Sea salt & pepper

Directions:

1. Heat a clean empty large skillet with olive oil over medium heat until the oil is hot.

2. Stir celery, garlic, and onion into the skillet and cook for about six minutes or until it is tender.

3. Add the remaining ingredients (except the lettuce) to the skillet, stir well to combine.

4. Reduce the heat to low and simmer for about 20 minutes to allow the sauce to thicken.

5. Spoon the mixture into the lettuce wraps and serve!

Spicy Lime Wings

Yield: 6 servings

Serving Size: ½ lb. wings

Prep Time: 5 min.

Cook Time: 35 min.

Ingredients:

For the Wings:

¼ c. sugar-free maple syrup

½ c. Thai chili paste

2 tbsp. rice wine vinegar

2 tbsp. soy sauce

3 lb. chicken wings, separated at the joints

For the Dipping Sauce:

¼ c. mayonnaise

1 tbsp. lime juice, fresh

$^{1/3}$ c. Greek yogurt, full fat, plain

Sea salt & pepper to taste

Directions:

1. In a large clean empty mixing bowl, combine the maple syrup, chili paste, vinegar, and soy sauce and whisk thoroughly.

2. Toss the wings in the cause and cover.

3. Chill for about 3 hours to allow the marinade to work.

4. Preheat the oven to 400° Fahrenheit and line a baking sheet with non-stick foil.

5. Place the wings onto the baking sheet, ensuring that they're not overlapping.

6. Bake the wings for 30 minutes, flipping them over halfway through to ensure even cooking and crispness.

7. Place wings under the broiler for 3-4 minutes until they're nice and brown.

8. In a clean empty small bowl, whisk together the ingredients for the dipping sauce.

9. Serve the wings hot with chilled dipping sauce!

Tex Mex Casserole

Yield: 8 servings

Serving Size: 1 square

Prep Time: 10 min.

Cook Time: 50 min.

Ingredients:

For the Crust:

1 c. mozzarella cheese, shredded

2 c. almond flour

2 oz. cream cheese, softened

3 lg. eggs, beaten

3 tsp. baking powder

For the Filling:

½ c. beef broth

1 c. cheddar cheese, shredded

1 tbsp. chili powder

1 tbsp. cumin, ground

1 tsp. garlic powder

1 tsp. paprika

2 lb. ground beef

2 tbsp. tomato paste

For the Topping:

Sour cream

Green onions, thinly sliced

Directions:

1. Preheat the oven to 350° Fahrenheit and grease a casserole or baking dish with non-stick spray or your preferred fat source.

2. In a clean food processor, combine all the ingredients for the crust and pulse until a thick batter is formed.

3. Pour the obtained batter into the baking dish and spread it out along the bottom, pushing it up on the sides. Set aside.

4. Heat a clean large skillet over medium-high heat and warm some oil in it.

5. Brown the beef and break it up as you do so.

6. Add beef broth, seasonings, and tomato paste into the skillet and stirr. Once completely combined, pour the mixture over the batter in the baking dish.

7. Bake for 35 to 40 minutes.

8. Remove the dish from the oven, top with cheese, then return it to the oven for another 5 to 10 minutes, or until the cheese is nice and bubbly.

9. Let stand for 10 minutes.

10. Serve topped with sour cream and guacamole if desired!

Chili Dog Casserole

Yield: 8 servings

Serving Size: 1 square

Prep Time: 15 min.

Cook Time: 50 min.

Ingredients:

½ tsp. celery salt
1 c. cheddar cheese, shredded

1 c. low-carb tomato sauce

1 c. water

1 lb. ground beef

1 sm. red bell pepper, diced

1 sm. yellow onion, diced

1 tbsp. chili powder

1 tsp. cumin, ground

1 tsp. Worcestershire sauce

2 cloves garlic, minced

2 tbsp. tomato paste

8 hotdogs, halved lengthwise

Sea salt & pepper to taste

Directions:

1. Preheat the oven to 400° Fahrenheit and grease a baking dish with non-stick spray or your preferred source of fat.

2. Evenly layer the hotdog halves along the bottom of the baking dish and set it aside.

3. In a large skillet over medium heat, let the oil heat up.

4. Once the oil is hot, combine peppers, onions, ground beef, and garlic. Cook until the beef is completely browned and make sure to break the beef into small chunks as you cook.

5. Into the skillet, pour tomato sauce, Worcestershire sauce, tomato paste, seasonings and water. Mix thoroughly and allow all ingredients to completely incorporate.

6. Heat the mixture so it boils and drop the heat to low. Simmer the content for about 30 minutes until the mixture gains a bit of thickness.

7. Spoon the chili onto the hotdogs in the baking dish and top with cheese.

8. Bake for about 20 minutes, or until warmed through and the cheese on top is bubbling to your preference.

9. Let cool for about ten minutes before cutting.

10. Serve hot and top with sour cream if desired!

Cheesy Meatball Bake

Yield: 8 servings

Serving Size: 4 balls

Prep Time: 15 min.

Cook Time: 45 min.

Ingredients:

½ c. parmesan cheese, grated

1 c. low-carb tomato sauce

1 c. mozzarella cheese, shredded

1 c. zucchini, shredded & pressed

1 lb. ground beef

1 lb. ground sausage

1 lg. egg

1 tbsp. garlic, minced

1 tsp. oregano, dried

2 c. provolone cheese, shredded

2 tsp. basil, dried

Sea salt & pepper to taste

Directions:

1. Preheat the oven to 400° Fahrenheit and grease a baking dish with non-stick spray or your preferred source of fat.

2. Place shredded zucchini into a kitchen towel or paper towel and press all the excess moisture from it.

3. In a large mixing bowl, combine zucchini, ground beef, ground sausage, egg, seasonings, mozzarella, and parmesan. Mix until completely combined.

4. Out of the mixture, make 32 meatballs and arrange them in one even layer in the baking dish.

5. Pour the tomato sauce into the baking dish, over the meatballs and sprinkle the provolone cheese on top.

6. Place in the oven to bake for 30 minutes.

7. Drain the excess liquid from the baking dish and return to oven.

8. Bake for another 10 to 15 minutes, or until cheese is bubbly and brown.

9. Serve hot!

Palak Paneer

Servings: 4

Time Required: About 10 minutes

Ingredients:

- 1 lb. fresh spinach
- 1 ½ cups paneer
- 2 tsp. olive oil
- 5 cloves garlic, minced
- 1 Tbsp. fresh ginger, peeled and minced
- 1 onion, chopped
- 2 tomatoes, chopped
- 2 tsp. ground cumin
- ½ tsp. cayenne pepper
- 2 tsp. garam masala
- 1 tsp. turmeric
- 1 tsp. salt
- ½ cup water

Directions:

1. Heat the oil in a large, heavy skillet over medium-high heat. When the oil is hot, add the garlic and ginger and sauté just until fragrant comes out for about 30 seconds.

2. Add the rest of the ingredients, excluding the paneer, and stir to combine well.

3. Sautee until the spinach is wilted and the spices are fragrant, about 4-5 minutes.

4. Carefully add the paneer to the pot, stirring gently to combine.

5. Serve hot.

Cauliflower Curry

Servings: 4-6

Time Required: About 30 minutes

Ingredients:

- 1 head cauliflower, chopped
- ½ onion, chopped
- 2 tomatoes, chopped
- 6 cloves garlic, minced
- 1 Tbsp. fresh ginger, peeled and minced
- ½ jalapeno chili, diced
- 1 tsp. olive oil
- ½ tsp. turmeric
- 1 tsp. ground cumin
- ½ tsp. garam masala
- ¾ tsp. salt
- ½ tsp. paprika

Directions:

1. Place onion, tomato, chili, ginger and garlic in a blender or food processor and blend until smooth.
2. Heat the oil in a large skillet over medium-high heat. When the oil is hot, add mixture from the blender to the pan.
3. Add the spices to the pan and stir to mix. Simmer for 5 minutes.
4. Stir the cauliflower into the pan and simmer until tender, about 15 minutes.
5. Serve hot.

Green Chili Cheese Bake

Servings: 4

Time Required: About 35 minutes

Ingredients:

- 4 eggs, beaten
- 1 cup half and half
- 10 oz. canned green chilis
- ½ tsp. salt
- ½ tsp. ground cumin
- 1 cup Monterey Jack cheese, grated
- ¼ cup fresh cilantro, chopped

Directions:

1. Preheat oven to 350 degrees Fahrenheit.
2. In a medium bowl, combine eggs, half and half, chilis, cheese, salt and cumin.
3. Pour the mixture into a greased baking pan. Cover the pan with aluminum foil.
4. Place the pan on the oven's center rack and bake until the egg is set, about 25-30 minutes.
5. Remove the pan from the pot and allow to cool slightly before serving.

Indian-Style Eggplant

Servings: 4

Time Required: About 30 minutes

Ingredients:

- 1 medium eggplant, peeled and sliced
- 1/3 cup olive oil
- 3 cloves garlic, minced
- ½ onion, chopped
- ¼ tsp. turmeric
- 1/8 tsp. cayenne pepper
- ½ tsp. salt
- 1/3 cup tomatoes, diced
- ½ cup water
- 2 Tbsp. fresh cilantro, chopped

Directions:

1. Heat 2 tablespoons of the olive oil in a large, heavy skillet. Once the oil is hot, add enough eggplant slices to cover the bottom of the pot liner. Allow the eggplant to brown well on the bottom, and add more eggplant as the slices shrink. Add more oil as necessary.

2. When the eggplant is browned and softened, add the onions and sauté for 5 minutes more.

3. Add the garlic and sauté for another minute.

4. Add the turmeric, cayenne, and salt. Sauté until fragrant, about a minute.

5. Add the tomatoes and water, and stir to combine everything in the pan.

6. Bring to a simmer and cook until the eggplant is fully cooked, about 15 minutes.

7. Transfer the eggplant and sauce to a serving platter.

8. Serve hot, garnished with cilantro.

Keto Pizza

Servings: 4

Time Required: About 30 minutes

Ingredients:

- 6 oz. mozzarella cheese
- ½ cup almond flour
- 2 Tbsp. psyllium husk
- 2 Tbsp. cream cheese
- 2 Tbsp. Parmesan cheese
- 1 large egg
- 1 tsp. Italian seasoning
- ½ tsp. salt
- ½ tsp. pepper
- 4 oz. cheddar cheese, shredded
- 1 medium vine tomato
- ¼ cup sugar-free marinara Sauce
- 2/3 medium bell pepper
- 2 Tbsp. fresh basil, chopped

Directions:

1. Preheat oven to 400 degrees Fahrenheit.

2. Combine almond flour, psyllium husk, parmesan cheese, Italian seasoning, salt, and pepper in a large mixing bowl.

3. Put mozzarella cheese is a microwave-safe bowl and microwave about 1 minute until it is soft. Remove from microwave and place cream cheese on top of the mozzarella in the bowl.

4. Stir egg into the dry ingredients in the mixing bowl. Add the heated cheeses to the bowl and mix thoroughly to create a dough.

5. Divide the dough into two equal portions and roll them out into a ¼-inch-thick crust on a lightly greased baking sheet.

6. Put the baking sheet into the oven and bake until the dough is just beginning to brown, about 10 minutes.

7. Remove the crust from the oven and allow to cool slightly.

8. Spread 2 tablespoons of marinara sauce on each pizza and top with 2 ounces cheddar cheese and chopped bell pepper.

9. Return the pizzas to the oven and bake for another 8-10 minutes.

10. Remove from the oven and serve hot.

Spaghetti Squash

Servings: 4

Time Required: About 60 minutes

Ingredients:

- 1 spaghetti squash, medium

Directions:

1. Preheat oven to 400 degrees Fahrenheit.

2. With a sharp knife, carefully cut the squash in half crosswise, across the short length of the squash instead of along the longer axis.

3. Place the squash halves on a baking sheet, cut side down.

4. Place the baking sheet on the oven's center rack and roast until the squash is tender, about 45-50 minutes.

5. Remove the squash and, while it's still hot, carefully shred the flesh into spaghetti-like strands with a fork.

6. Serve the squash hot with butter.

Steamed Artichokes

Servings: 4

Time Required: About 40 minutes

Ingredients:

- 4 artichokes, medium-sized
- 1 lemon
- 4 cups vegetable stock
- ¼ tsp. kosher salt

Directions:

1. Trim the artichoke stems to an inch in length. Trim the other end of the artichokes, too, cutting the inch from the ends of the leaves. Discard the trimmings.
2. Slice the lemon into four slices.
3. Place the steamer rack into the steamer pot and place the lemon slices on the rack. Place the artichokes, stem end up, on the lemon slices, one artichoke on each lemon slice.
4. Pour the stock carefully into the pot. Season with salt.
5. Cover the pot.
6. Steam until the artichokes are tender, about 25-35 minutes.
7. Serve the artichokes with melted butter for dipping.

Cheesy Cauliflower Casserole

Servings: 4-6

Time Required: About 60 minutes

Ingredients:

- 1 head cauliflower
- 2 eggs
- 2 Tbsp. heavy cream
- 2 oz. cream cheese
- ½ cup sour cream
- ½ cup Parmesan cheese, grated
- 1 cup cheddar cheese, grated
- 2 Tbsp. butter
- 1 cup water

Directions:

1. Preheat oven to 350 degrees Fahrenheit.

2. Add eggs, cream, sour cream, cream cheese, parmesan and cheddar cheese to a blender or food processor. Blend to combine.

3. Add cauliflower to the food processor and blend, pulsing so that you can stop when the mixture is still chunky, not smooth.

4. Grease a casserole pan and pour the mixture into the pan.

5. Place the pan on the oven's center rack and bake until the casserole is bubbly, about 45 minutes.

6. Remove the pan and serve the casserole hot.

Thai-Style Zucchini Noodles

Servings: 3

Time Required: About 25 minutes

Ingredients:

- 2 medium zucchini, spiralized
- ½ cup sliced mushrooms
- 1 cup shredded broccoli slaw mix
- 1 tsp. sesame oil
- ¼ cup almond butter
- 2 Tbsp. soy sauce
- 2 Tbsp. sesame oil
- ¼ tsp. garlic powder
- 1 tsp. crushed red pepper flakes
- 1 tsp. sugar-free sweetener

Directions:

1. Heat sesame oil in a large skillet on medium heat. Add the shredded broccoli slaw mix and mushrooms, sautéing until the vegetables have softened.

2. Cut zucchini noodles using a vegetable spiralizer or a vegetable peeler. Press the noodles between paper towels to remove some of their moisture.

3. Heat the noodles in the skillet, stirring often, until they're soft but not mushy, about 3-5 minutes.

4. Combine the rest of the ingredients in a small mixing bowl and whisk together. Adjust the consistency with water if necessary to make a sauce.

5. Divide the noodles evenly between three serving bowls and top with the
   sauce.

Keto Italian-Style Dumplings

Servings: 5

Time Required: About 30 minutes

Ingredients:

For dough:

- 2 cups almond flour
- 2 cups mozzarella cheese, shredded
- ¼ cup butter
- 1 large egg
- 1 large egg yolk

For sauce:

- ¼ cup salted butter
- 1 tsp. lemon zest
- 1 tsp. fresh thyme leaves

Directions:

1. Combine the mozzarella cheese and butter in a microwave-safe bowl and microwave for 1 minute. Stir and then microwave for another minute. Stir thoroughly and allow to cool.

2. Stir in egg yolk, then stir in the almond flour to make a dough.

3. Transfer the dough to a clean, smooth surface and knead until the dough is stretchy. Shape the dough into a roll about an inch in diameter. Slice the roll into pieces about ½-inch thick.

4. Pop the dough pieces into the freezer for about 10 minutes to make them more firm.

5. Bring a large pot of water to a boil and carefully add the dumplings. Cook them for 1-2 minutes and then carefully remove them with a slotted spoon.

6. Melt the butter in a skillet, then add the thyme and lemon zest, stirring for about 2 minutes.

7. Gently add the dumplings to the pan and stir to coat with the sauce.

8. Season to taste with salt and pepper and serve hot.

Golden Eggplant Fries

Servings: 6

Time Required: About 60 minutes

Ingredients:

- 2 large eggplants
- 2 eggs
- ½ cup coconut flour
- ½ cup Parmesan cheese, grated
- ½ tsp. garlic powder
- 1/8 tsp. salt
- 1/8 tsp. pepper
- ½ tsp. parsley flakes
- ½ cup olive oil

Directions:

1. Peel the eggplant and cut into strips about 1 inch wide and 3 inches long.
2. Beat the 2 eggs in a small bowl.
3. Combine the Parmesan cheese, coconut flour, garlic powder, salt, pepper and parsley flakes in a medium bowl.
4. Heat the oil in a skillet over medium-high heat.
5. Dip the eggplant pieces in the egg, then dredge in the cheese mixture.
6. Fry the eggplant in the hot oil until it's golden brown, turning once to brown both sides.
7. Transfer to a paper towel to soak up excess oil, and then serve hot.

Mashed Cauliflower

Servings: 4-6

Time Required: About 20 minutes

Ingredients:

- 1 head cauliflower
- 1/8 tsp. salt
- 1/8 tsp. freshly ground black pepper
- ¼ tsp. garlic powder
- 1 cup water

Directions:

1. Chop the cauliflower coarsely and discard the tough core.
2. Place a steamer rack in a steamer pot and add a cup of water.
3. Place the cauliflower on top of the steamer rack.
4. Steam until the cauliflower is tender, about 15 minutes.
5. Carefully drain the water and remove the steamer rack, returning the cauliflower to the pot once it's drained.
6. If you have an immersion blender, use it to blend the cauliflower to a smooth puree, adding the seasonings as you blend. If you don't have an immersion blender, transfer the cauliflower to a blender or food processor. Optionally, you can add a tablespoon of butter as you blend for a creamier consistency.
7. Serve hot.

Crispy Broccoli Nuggets

Servings: 4-6

Time Required: About 25 minutes

Ingredients:

- ¾ cup almond flour
- 7 Tbsp. flaxseed meal
- 4 oz. fresh broccoli
- 4 oz. mozzarella cheese
- 2 large eggs
- 2 tsp. baking powder
- Salt and pepper to taste
- ¼ cup mayonnaise
- ¼ cup fresh chopped dill
- ½ Tbsp. lemon juice

Directions:

1. Add broccoli to a food processor and pulse until the broccoli is ground to a meal-like consistency.
2. Combine the cheese, almond flour, flaxseed meal and baking powder with the broccoli in a large mixing bowl.
3. Add the eggs and mix well. to form a thick batter
4. Form the batter into 1-inch balls and dredge in flax seed meal.
5. Heat cooking oil in a fryer or deep skillet to 375 degrees Fahrenheit.
6. Fry the nuggets until they're golden brown, turning once to brown both side. This should take 3-5 minutes.
7. Serve hot.

www.ingramcontent.com/pod-product-compliance
Lightning Source LLC
Chambersburg PA
CBHW081317250726
48662CB00008B/2611